Habit Hacking

Rewiring Your Brain for Success

Cedric E. Warren

Table of Contents

We are what we repeatedly do. Excellence, then,
is not an act, but a habit.

Chapter 1. Introduction

Unlock the potential of your mind and embrace the power of habit with our Special Report on Habit Hacking: Rewiring Your Brain for Success. This isn't your typical scientific discourse on neuroplasticity and brain diagrams. Instead, this is a user-friendly, empowering guide that delves into practical steps and novel strategies to recalibrate your habit formation for optimal success. The journey to greatness doesn't have to be tedious, and this refreshing report is the enthusiastic cheerleader you've needed, making the process exciting, engaging, and genuinely enjoyable. Get ready to elevate your life to new heights because success is not solely about talent or luck—it's about shaping your habits. Join us on this guided expedition to penetrate the layers of your habits and hack them to work in your favor! Purchase this Special Report today, and put yourself on a fast track towards success.

Chapter 2. Understanding the Power of Habits

Behavioral scientists, psychologists, and the most successful people around us all underscore the importance of habits. Actually, our habits are powerful tools that can define our success, happiness, wellbeing, or sadly, our failure—it all depends on the nature of the habits we form. Later in this chapter, we will delve deeper into the true power of habits utilizing examples from everyday life and a rich base of research.

2.1. The Habit Loop: Cue, Routine, and Reward

At the most basic level, habits can be understood as a three-step loop that includes a cue, a routine, and a reward. Let's break it down:

1. *Cue*: The cue is a trigger that tells your brain to go into automatic mode and initiates the routine. It can be anything— a location, a time of day, an emotional state, the presence of particular people, or just a proceeding action.

2. *Routine*: This is the actual habituated behavior or sequence of actions that you automatically carry out once you've been cued. It could be physical, mental, or emotional.

3. *Reward*: Last, but not least, the reward. This is the positive reinforcement that your brain gets after the routine. This reward could be something as substantial as a feeling of satisfaction, a taste of your favorite food, a round of applause, a sense of accomplishment, or even relief from discomfort.

This "habit loop" is a self-reinforcing cycle - a neurological loop that governs any habit. It's how our brain economizes our thinking and actions, saving our cognitive energy for more important decisions.

2.2. The Influence of Habits on Daily Life

Habits frame a larger part of our daily life than most of us realize. They are at work from the moment we wake up until we retire for the day. They influence the decisions we make, the routines we follow, and consequently, the results we achieve in life.

Our morning routine—wake up, brush our teeth, take a shower, have breakfast—is nothing but a series of habits. We effortlessly glide through these activities, almost on autopilot, without having to put any conscious thought into executing them. This effortless automation is the reason habits are so important; they influence our lives subtly yet persistently.

The autopilot nature of habits is why they can be powerful drivers of success and productivity. Imagine if every task required cognitive effort—you'd exhaust your cognitive resources before you got halfway through your day! But when routines become habits, they become second nature. It saves energy and time, allowing us to focus on complex tasks and problems.

2.3. Habits and Success: An Inextricable Connection

The essence of success isn't grand, radical changes. It's found instead in the seemingly inconsequential, day-to-day habits. It's the incremental improvements, the tiny changes we make each day that accumulate into substantial gains over time. That's where habits play an indelible role.

Achieving success is often about embracing better habits and jettisoning the ones that are holding you back. Successful people do not just work harder; they work better, thanks to a system of powerful habits that guide their everyday life. For instance, regular reading is a simple habit that enhances knowledge and cognitive function—traits synonymous with numerous successful individuals.

However, success isn't solely about professional accomplishments. It's also about personal growth and emotional well-being. It's about growing as a human being, enhancing your knowledge, understanding yourself better, and achieving peace of mind. And all these different facets of success are deeply connected to the habits we cultivate.

2.4. Transforming your life One Habit at a Time

The power of habits lies not in individual habits but in the cumulative impact of all our habits. Habits are interlocking, creating a structure that shapes our entire lives. For the same reason, habit change creates a ripple effect. Even small changes can have a big overarching impact on our lives, sometimes in areas seemingly unrelated to the habit itself.

Research has shown that when people start habitually exercising, even as infrequently as once a week, they start changing other, unrelated patterns in their lives, often unknowingly. Typically, people who exercise start eating healthier food, reducing their caffeine intake, curbing excessive alcohol consumption, and even using their credit cards less.

Author's note: The transformational power of habits is truly staggering. By shaping our habits, we can completely transform the architecture of our everyday life and, eventually, our destiny.

By this point, you should feel a growing awareness of the sheer influence your habits have on your life. In our upcoming chapters, you will learn how to decode your existing habits, some foolproof strategies to install beneficial habits, and practical ways to circumvent any roadblocks that you encounter on your habit formation journey. You are essentially just a few habit changes away from the success you desire and deserve. Remember, your habits, regardless of how small they seem, cast a long shadow over your future. Let's learn how to cast the right shadows!

Chapter 3. The Neuroscience behind Habits: A User-friendly Explanation

The neurological landscape within our brain is a prodigious expanse where myriad activities are conducted. Understanding it doesn't require you to hold an advanced degree in neurobiology, it just needs a user-friendly frame of reference to simplify the complex latticework of our cognitive function. Let's make our foray into the neural domain where habits are formed and sustained.

3.1. Habit Loops and the Rat Race: A Simple Introduction

To appreciate the neuroscience behind habits, it's beneficial to first grasp the concept of habit loops. Think of these loops as the brain's simplified instructions for habitual actions—like autopilot. Imagine a rat in a maze. At first, the creature scampers around, bumping into walls, sniffing at dead ends, desperately in search of the delicious piece of cheese placed in one corner. Initially, the rat's brain is in overdrive, firing neurons to encode this newfound information. Soon, a mental pattern or 'shortcut' begins to form. The rat will learn the easiest path to the cheese, creating a habit loop and cementing its actions into habituated responses.

3.2. The Triad of Habit Formation: Cue, Routine, and Reward

Every habit loop has three integral components: a cue, a routine, and a reward. The cue is what prompts the habit to start. The routine is the behavior itself. The reward, as you might guess, is the benefit or payoff that the brain receives from carrying out the routine. Understanding this triad is crucial for comprehending habit formation as it is the fulcrum on which our behaviors pivot.

Cue: It triggers the brain to initiate a routine. It's a spark that lights the fire. From the smell of coffee brewing that leads you to your morning mug to the buzz of your phone that makes you check your notifications, cues are everywhere.

Routine: This is the action conducted in response to the cue. It's the meat of the habit—what we often think of as the habit itself.

Reward: This is the payoff that reinforces the habit loop. The brain identifies the patterns that provide a rewards and prioritizes them for future identification and replication, perpetuating the habit loop.

3.3. Neuroplasticity: The Reason Why Habits Stick

An essential concept in the understanding of habit formation is neuroplasticity. Our brain is not the rigid, unchangeable organ we used to believe it to be. Its structure and functionality are malleable, meaning they can reshape and reorganize themselves based on behavioral activation. It's plastic at a neurological level. Repetitive or prominent behaviors can physically rewire the circuitry of your brain.

In the context of habits, neuroplasticity refers to the brain's ability to form new neural connections and pathways as a result of repetitive behavior. When you conduct a routine regularly, it effectively fortifies the neural pathways associated with it, making it easier for your brain to trigger the same pattern in the future. This explains why habitual actions can be conducted effortlessly and often unconsciously. Certain parts of your brain related to the habit become more efficient, strengthening the connections between neurons and facilitating faster, smoother information processing.

3.4. Habit-forming Regions of the Brain

The basal ganglia and the prefrontal cortex are two key players in the habit formation process. The basal ganglia, situated deep within the brain, are involved in a variety of complex functions, including voluntary motor control, procedural learning, and habit formation. In contrast, the prefrontal cortex, located at the very front of the brain, is involved in planning complex cognitive behavior, personality expression, decision making, and moderating social behavior- "executive functions."

When you're learning something new, your prefrontal cortex is hard at work assimilating all the new information. Once it becomes a routine, the basal ganglia take over, reducing the cognitive load and freeing up the prefrontal cortex for other tasks. This dual-system is what enables you to do things 'on autopilot,' like driving to work while planning your day or brushing your teeth while musing about your breakfast menu.

3.5. A Call to Frequency – The Power of Repetition

Repetition amplifies the process of habit formation. As mentioned earlier, with every repetition of a behavior, the corresponding neural pathway strengthens. This interaction fosters efficiency, and gradually the behavior requires less effort and becomes almost automatic. This reduced mental effort can be linked to the concept of "Hebb's law" or "neurons that fire together, wire together." It's our brain's natural mechanism to seek out and reinforce beneficial behavior patterns. However, keep in mind that what the brain perceives as rewarding might not always be in our best long-term interest. The same law can apply to destructive habits like smoking, binge eating, or procrastinating.

By understanding the user-friendly neuroscience behind habits, we can take charge of our habit loops, leverage the power of neuroplasticity, capitalize on the dual-process theory, and harness the strengthening effects of repetition to deliberately forge beneficial habits. Metaphorically, our brain is clay in our hands, ready to be molded into patterns that can fuel our success. In the upcoming chapters, we'll delve deeper into how you can use this knowledge to decode your existing habits and craft new ones that lead you to your desired success.

Chapter 4. Decoding Your Existing Habits: The Self-Audit

To begin your journey into optimizing your habit formation, it's essential to conduct a thorough self-audit of your existing habits. This process will provide you with a clear map on which potential changes to address and what habit patterns to focus on. So, brace yourself for an expedition into your lifestyle, your daily routine, your thought progression, and, most importantly, your subconscious habits.

4.1. Uncovering the Patterns

The first step toward understanding your habits is uncovering the patterns that govern your life. To a surprising extent, our lives are largely a result of recurring cycles. Whether it's the daily morning routine having a cup of coffee, reading the newspaper, and then heading out for a jog, or the bi-weekly pattern of paying bills or having a family dinner, patterns are omnipresent.

Make a list of your daily routines, both explicit, like the morning routine, and implicit, like absent-mindedly checking your phone during work breaks. It's usually the unconscious habits you're not aware of that hold the most transformative potential. Utilizing a habit journal for a week or a even month can be a useful tool to document all activities conducted during an entire day.

As continuous observation is essential at this stage, remember to be patient with yourself. Habits, particularly subconscious ones, cannot be identified and thoroughly understood in a matter of days.

4.2. Categorize Your Habits

Once you have scrutinized your daily and weekly routines and recorded all of your observed habits, the next step is to categorize them. This categorization primarily involves classifying them as beneficial, neutral, or harmful.

Beneficial habits are those that are clearly contributing to your physical, emotional, and mental well-being and are steering you towards your life objectives. These can range from having a balanced breakfast, engaging in regular exercise, to dedicating a specific part of the day to self-study or honing a skill.

Neutral habits are actions that don't significantly add to or detract from your quality of life, such as having a favorite spot to sit in at home, or listening to the news while driving. These habits may well occupy a substantial part of our day, yet their effect on our life trajectory is minimal.

Harmful habits are those activities that are potentially destructive, stifling your progress towards achieving your goals and may wreak havoc on your health and wellbeing. These might include overindulging in alcohol, procrastination, or fostering toxic relationships.

By grouping your habits according to their prospective impacts, you can gain precious insight into how your daily actions might be shaping your life.

4.3. The Cause and Effect

Now we move on to a more nuanced analysis – identifying the triggers and effects of each habit. Every habit has a prompt, an action, and a reward. This structure is referred to as the habit loop. The prompt triggers the habit, the reward reinforces it, and the loop continues.

Take each habit and note its trigger, routine, and reward. For example, if you have the habit of biting your nails when you're nervous (trigger), the action is the nail-biting, and the reward could be a temporary relief from nervousness.

Knowing the components of the habit loop is significant, as it reduces the formerly overwhelming task of changing a habit to the relatively simpler task of identifying and modifying its components.

4.4. Time Taken and Frequency

Understanding the frequency and time taken by each habit is also extremely crucial. Some habits may occur daily, while others may occur weekly or even monthly. Moreover, some habits occur multiple times a day. They may seem insignificant, but when added up, they can amount to a substantial chunk of your daily routine. It also relates to the energy spent and the opportunity cost associated with each action.

The comprehensive self-audit method described here will significantly augment your understanding of your existing habits. And, per the adage, 'knowledge is power', this newfound understanding of your patterns will prove to be an immensely powerful tool in reshaping and retuning your habits, enabling you to curate a lifestyle that most aligns with your aspirations.

Bear in mind, this self-audit is not a one-off process, but something to be revisited and updated on a regular basis as your habits, endeavors, and circumstances evolve. Continuous introspection will yield the best results in your habit hacking journey. So, remain observant, stay patient, and keep adjusting as per the insight garnered from this self-audit process.

Chapter 5. Roadblocks to Success: Bad Habits and How to Identify Them

The journey to success, unfortunately, is not always on a direct route, nor is it free of inconveniences. One of the most significant impediments on this journey arises from our bad or counterproductive habits. Simply put, bad habits are those ingrained behaviors that, when carried out consistently, contrarily affect our wellbeing or hinder our progress toward our desired goals. Now, let's take a deeper look into exactly what stands in our way and draw a road map for identifying these detrimental habits.

5.1. Understanding Bad Habits

Many of us grapple with the pernicious effects of bad habits every day, from inordinate procrastination to constantly misplacing our keys. These behaviors, in spite of their negative consequences on our health, productivity or tranquility, intermittently persist, often fueled by psychological cravings or as coping mechanisms to stress or anxiety.

Bad habits come in many shapes and forms. Some are fairly evident, such as smoking, excessive drinking, unhealthy eating, or obsessively biting your nails. Others are more subtle, like perfectionism, constant lateness, chronic negativity, impulse shopping, or even excessive screen time. Whatever form they take, they invariably disrupt your life in one way or another, and only by identifying them can we begin the process of change.

5.2. The Science behind Bad Habits

Before diving into the process of identifying bad habits, it is instructive to understand the science behind them. Bad habits, like their good counterparts, are essentially birthed from the brain's inherent nature to automate repeated behaviors, thus conserving energy for more vital tasks. This process of habituation forms the basis of all habits. The more we engage in a specific behavior, the more ingrained it becomes, facilitated by the strengthening of specific neural pathways.

In relation to bad habits, stress and boredom are often key players in their formation. Owing to the brain's reward system, coping mechanisms that provide immediate, albeit temporary, relief from negative emotions are prone to become habitual. Regrettably, these 'quick-fix' solutions often lead to long-term detriment.

5.3. Recognizing Your Bad Habits

Observation and introspection are two crucial steps in identifying your bad habits. Begin by reflecting on your daily routines. What actions do you repeat daily without conscious thought? You might notice obvious bad habits, like scrolling on your phone for hours or reaching for unhealthy snacks when stressed.

Next, consider the less glaring, yet potentially harmful habits. Are you consistently late to appointments or work, causing stress or damage to relationships or professional reputation? Are you perpetually in a state of worry about the future? Are you neglecting physical activity? Successful identification goes beyond the noticeable and requires a comprehensive, honest examination of your behaviors.

5.4. Analyzing the Impact of Bad Habits

Once a list of potential bad habits has been drawn up, the next step is to evaluate their impact on your life. Consider the implications of these actions on your physical health, emotional wellbeing, productivity, relationships, career, and overall life goals. This analysis encourages a deeper awareness of the severity of your habits, further motivating you to instigate changes.

5.5. Establishing Triggers for Your Bad Habits

Identifying triggers is a fundamental step in understanding your bad habits. Triggers are circumstances or situations that illicit the execution of a particular habit. It could be an emotional state, a particular time, a place, another person, or even previously established habits. For example, you might find you binge on sweets after a stressful day at work, or waste time on social media after waking up.

The journey of identifying and understanding your bad habits takes patience and self-awareness. It is a treacherous path to tread, strewn with moments of self-conflict and realization. Yet, the reward at the end—a better, more successful version of you—is indeed worth the struggle. With this knowledge, you can understand the anatomy of your bad habits, allowing you to strategically dismantle them and commence the next phase of your journey: crafting beneficial habits.

Chapter 6. The Art of Crafting Beneficial Habits

Understanding the significance of habits is simply the first step of our comprehensive guide. However, furthermore, being able to craft beneficial habits for yourself is where this journey truly begins to take shape.

6.1. Fundamental Principles

Before diving into the intricate details of shaping beneficial habits, it is crucial to understand some fundamental principles. We are not just manually producing habits out of thin air; we're invoking a genuine change emanating from deep within us. So, what does this require of us? Here are three guiding principles:

1. Insight: Before proceeding, you should have a thorough understanding of your behaviors, tendencies, and routines. Acknowledging the habits you wish to create and understanding how they impact your life are vital in determining the strength of your commitment to them.

2. Consistency: This principle champions the motto, "frequency over quantity." Regardless of the scope of your routine, being consistent with it holds more weight in achieving results. Small incremental steps, when done consistently, yield significant results over time.

3. Patience: Rome wasn't built in a day, right? So, understanding that genuine change is something cultivated over time is essential. Tolerating discomfort and accepting the iterative nature of the process are pertinent traits of patience in this context.

6.2. Identifying Beneficial Habits

The idea of beneficial habits might vary from individual to individual due to the diversity in personal goals and preferred lifestyles. However, commonalities exist among these habits, which tend to promote general wellbeing.

Some examples of broadly beneficial habits include daily exercise, maintaining a balanced diet, practicing mindfulness, keeping a gratitude journal, implementing a regular sleeping routine, continuously learning, and networking.

These habits, when tailored specifically to your personal and professional objectives, become the foundation upon which you build your success.

6.3. Define Clear Goals

When crafting beneficial habits, it's vital to ensure that you have clear, well-defined goals. This is where SMART goals come into play. Based on this, habits should be:

- Specific – Define your habits in the clearest of terms, leaving no ambiguity. Instead of saying "I want to read more," say "I want to read for 30 minutes each day."

- Measurable – Have some metric or key performance indicator to track your progress. In the example above, 30 minutes is our measurable metric.

- Achievable – Ensure the habit is practical and attainable considering your resources and constraints. It would be unreasonable to think you can read an entire book every day.

- Relevant – The habit must align with your larger life goals. If you're an entrepreneur, reading business books could be more pertinent to your success than reading fantasy novels.

- Time-bound – Every habit should have a realistic timeline which bestows urgency and aids in preventing procrastination.

6.4. Implementing Habit Stacking and Pairing

Habit Stacking, popularized by productivity expert James Clear in "Atomic Habits," adopts a simple trick: after completing an existing habit, enforce a new habit. For example, after brushing your teeth (existing habit), you could practice five minutes of mindfulness (new habit).

On a similar note, habit pairing involves combining a new habit you want to develop with a current habit that you enjoy. Suppose you love drinking coffee each morning. You could pair this with reading for 15 minutes, thus making the new habit more enjoyable and, therefore, easier to maintain.

6.5. Dealing with Resistance

Resistance is part of the journey of creating new habits. Your brain prefers comfort and routine, and creating new habits means pushing past the boundaries of your comfort zone. To help in this area, use visualization. Picture the rewards that come with the habit and the end results. It is also important to break down the habit into the smallest possible steps to make it seem doable – this tactic is popularly known as Kaizen, or "continuous improvement."

6.6. Leverage the Power of Accountability

Seeking accountability could also help significantly in crafting beneficial habits. Whether it's a friend, a coach, or a mentor, having someone monitor your progress makes you more likely to persist. You are more likely to stick with new habits when you know someone else is watching. This also includes accountability to oneself through maintaining an open and updated habit tracker.

Through understanding the art of crafting beneficial habits, we learn that creating these habits is not an act of mere discipline or determination, but it's a balanced blend of self-awareness, systematic approach, patience, consistency, and a dash of creativity. We are not just instilling rote routines in our day; we are indeed hacking our brains to create lasting lifestyle changes. By internalizing these practices, you equip yourself with the power to change any aspect of your life and character, stepping towards becoming the best version of yourself.

Chapter 7. The Science of Habit Formation: Consistency and Time Frame

In the labyrinth of habits, the journey toward creating new, beneficial ones is a refined science. It orbits around the guiding principles of consistency and the hardness of a time frame, two pillars that uphold the architecture of habit formation.

7.1. The Principle of Consistency

Undeniably, consistency is the lifeblood of any habit. In the grand orchestra that is habit creation, it plays the role of the conductor, coordinating all elements and ensuring they function in harmonious unison.

It begins with a simple action executed repeatedly. Over time, this action leads to a strong neural pathway being formed in the brain, creating what we commonly understand as a habit.

Here's a detailed step-by-step process of how habits take shape through consistency.

1. Your brain encounters a new activity.

2. A neural pattern is created for this activity in the brain.

3. With repetition, the neural pattern becomes stronger, making the activity easier to perform.

4. As the action gets ingrained, less mental effort is required to do it, thus leading to automation. This action is now deemed a habit.

This process is the reason we keep keys in the same place, wake up at a specific time, or follow a particular routine at the gym.

7.2. How to Foster Consistency

Creating consistency is much like tending to a sapling. Here are some strategies to nurture this seed and allow it to grow into a mighty habit tree:

1. Find your 'why': The impulse to be consistent stems from understanding the importance of the end goal. Keeping that goal in sight can fuel your consistency. Root yourself to a strong 'why', and the 'how' will follow.

2. Start small: Break your desired habits into smaller, more achievable actions. These bite-sized portions are far less intimidating and easier to maintain consistency with over time.

3. Use a habit tracker: Monitoring progress can boost motivation and keep you committed. It tangibly embodies your progress, making consistency more rewarding.

4. Routine: Embed the new habit into your existing routine. We're more likely to stick to something if it fits seamlessly within our daily actions.

5. Regular rewards: Reinforcement can bolster motivation. Small rewards for consistency further enhances the desire to continue with the habit.

7.3. The Role of Time Frame

In tandem with consistency, the time frame plays an instrumental role in habit cultivation. While consistency provides the structure, the time frame supplies the boundaries within which the habit formation process thrives.

Many cultural references contribute to the popular belief that it takes 21 days to form a habit. Yet, newer scientific evidence, such as the study conducted by Phillipa Lally, a health psychology researcher at

University College London, illustrates that the average time to form a habit is actually closer to 66 days.

The variability, however, is significant, contingent upon the complexity of the habit and the individual's determination. It may take anywhere from 18 to 254 days!

7.4. Developing a Made-to-Measure Time Frame

There's no one-size-fits-all time frame for habit formation. The number of days it will take for an action to become automatic will differ from person to person and habit to habit. Here are few strategies to craft the perfect time frame for your habit:

1. Be realistic: Setting unattainable goals can lead to disappointment. Select a time frame you believe you can commit to for the duration of habit formation. Completion of the time frame enhances your trust and confidence in yourself.

2. Allow for flexibility: Life happens, derailing your plan from time to time. Allow some slack for unforeseen events.

3. Gradual increase: You may start with a short time frame and gradually increase it as you build both the habit and the confidence in the process.

4. Pair it with existing habits: It can be beneficial to pair the new habit with an existing habit which serves as a reminder to keep up with the habit creation process.

In the vast universe of habit hacking, the science of habit formation hinges largely on understanding and harnessing the power of consistency and the time frame. Through this dual mastery, you can ensure a sturdy bridge leading toward the creation of successful habits that will rewrite the narrative of your life for the better.

Chapter 8. Practical Strategies for Installing New Habits

Great habits are the foundation of a prosperous life. But the challenge often lies in building those highly effective habits in the first place. We've all been there – starting a new habit with a burst of enthusiasm, only to find it fizzles out after a few days or weeks. So, how do you go about making new habits stick? Our goal in this chapter is to provide some practical strategies specifically curated for you, to help you facilitate this journey toward installing new habits.

8.1. Understanding Your Motivations

Every habit formation journey starts with a heartfelt desire to make a change. What ignites that desire can be different for each person. It could be a need to elevate your lifestyle, manage your time more effectively or to build better relationships. Whatever the reason behind your intent to form a new habit, it is crucial to authentically identify and understand this motivation. This understanding becomes the fuel that powers your commitment to persist with the habit, especially during challenging phases.

8.2. Creating SMART Goals

One effective strategy for habit creation revolves around making your goals SMART: Specific, Measurable, Achievable, Relevant and Time-bound. Let's unpack these a little bit:

- Specific: Vague goals lack direction. Aim for habit goals that are clear and well-defined. Instead of "I want to read more", opt for "I want to read one book a month".

- Measurable: By making your goals measurable, you add a quantitative aspect that makes it easier to track your progress. "I will read for 30 minutes each day" is a measurable goal.

- Achievable: Aim high but stay grounded in practicality. Going from no reading to promising to finish a 500-page book in a week might not be achievable.

- Relevant: Your new habits should be aligned with your long-term goals and life vision. If reading science fiction doesn't excite you, then pushing for it won't help much in the long run.

- Time-bound: Having a time framework adds a sense of urgency and increases motivation. Specify "I will finish this book in two weeks".

8.3. Habit Stacking

Habit stacking is a powerful technique developed by productivity expert and author James Clear. The idea is to leverage the habits you already do consistently by pairing them with new habit(s) you are trying to build. By "stacking" them together, you create a chain of habits, where each habit acts as a cue for the next. This approach offers an already established platform (your existing habit) onto which you add your new habit, increasing the likelihood of consistency. Moreover, accomplishing these small wins can significantly boost your confidence and motivation.

8.4. Designing an Environment to Foster Habits

Your environment plays a significant role in nurturing or sabotaging your habits. If your environment is not conducive to your new habits, it might take more effort to stick to them. Identify any environmental blockers, and actively change them to support your new habits. For instance, if your goal is to drink more water, keep a water bottle at your desk to remind when you sit to work.

8.5. Leveraging Technology

Technology can be an asset while forming new habits. Countless habit-tracking apps, digital reminders and resources on the internet can provide structure and support needed to make the habit stick. Additionally, joining online communities such as forums or discussion groups that share similar habit goals can offer encouragement and inspiration.

8.6. Building Accountability

Accountability is the commitment glue that can bind you to your habit goals. This could be as simple as sharing your goals with a friend, hiring a coach, or joining a group with similar objectives. Knowing that someone will check up on your progress builds a sense of responsibility and increases the chances of persisting with your habit efforts.

8.7. Embracing Progress over Perfection

Finally, understand that the journey to installing a new habit is not always a linear one. There may be slippages and setbacks along the way, and that is perfectly okay. The objective is not to achieve perfection but to embrace progress. Celebrate your victories, however small they may be, as these are the stepping stones towards the ultimate vision of your successful self.

By applying these practical strategies, you increase your chances of creating habits that last. Eventually, you are not just installing new habits. Instead, you're paving a path towards becoming a better version of yourself. Remember, the journey to success begins with creating powerful habits. And with these strategies, you are equipped to traverse this journey with calculated planning and precision. Today marks the start of your transformation!

Chapter 9. Mind Hacks to Solidify Your New Habits

So, you've embarked on your journey towards habit hacking, meticulously curating beneficial habits and rigorously practicing them. Yet, you might find yourself falling short of making these habits second nature. Enter mind hacks - strategic psychological tools that can augment your effort in habit solidification. Leveraging an amalgam of neuroscience, psychology and personal development principles, these methods can tailor your mindset in a way that bolsters your habit practice, simultaneously instilling a sense of agency and ease in this process. Let's unravel some potent mind hacks that can be your trusty allies in solidifying your new habits.

9.1. Visualization

The power of visualization is an underplayed yet remarkably influential tool in the realm of habit formation. Often used by athletes and successful individuals, visualization uses the principle of neuroplasticity, the brain's ability to rewire itself. By vividly imagining performing a habit, from beginning to end, you are essentially training your brain to carry it out without physical practice.

Execute this by setting aside a quiet time daily to picture yourself carrying out each step of your new habit. For instance, if your new habit is reading nightly, imagine yourself picking up the book, flipping open to your bookmarked page, reading and placing it back on your bedside table. The key is to engage all your senses in this mental rehearsal - the texture of the book's cover in your hand, the rustling of the pages turning, the scent of the ink - all contribute to making the brain's neural connections stronger.

9.2. Positive Affirmations

Never underestimate the potency of your internal dialogue. What you repetitively say to yourself programs your subconscious mind and gradually transmutes into your automatic belief system and behavior. This principle can be harnessed to solidify new habits.

List out affirmations corresponding to your new habits. For instance, if your new habit is to quit smoking, an affirmation would be "I am effortlessly releasing the need for smoking; my lungs are regaining their health each day." Ensure your affirmations are positive, present tense, and personal. Consistently recite these to yourself, particularly during times you find your resolve to practice the habit waning.

9.3. Reward Mechanics

Our brains are wired to seek pleasure and satisfaction. Skillfully leveraging this characteristic can aid in the habit solidification process through a mechanism known as the 'habit loop', which consists of three parts: cue, routine, and reward. The 'reward' part not only provides a sense of pleasure post routine completion, but it also strengthens neural pathways involved in the habit, making subsequent practice easier.

Consider meaningful rewards that you can incorporate at the end of your habit routine. This doesn't necessarily have to be extravagant; even the simple act of savoring a cup of your favorite tea or indulging in a few minutes of solitude can serve the purpose.

9.4. Accountability Structures

The establishment of accountability, either to oneself or to someone else, can motivate us to consistently perform a new habit until it becomes an ingrained part of our routine. This can be as simple as maintaining a habit tracker journal or as social as making a pact with a companion who is also on a journey of habit formation.

Practicing these mind hacks, alongside being consistent with your habit formation techniques, can be a game-changer in the endeavor of solidifying your new habits. Remember, patience and perseverance are your best companions in this journey. As the famous saying goes, "It's not about where you start, but the direction in which you aim." So, continue in your pursuit of solidifying new habits, and let these mind tools guide you towards uncompromised success.

Chapter 10. Dealing with Potential Setbacks on Your Habit Hacking Journey

Any journey towards habit transformation is replete with potential obstacles, setbacks, and detours. The key to maintaining your trajectory towards success is understanding that these aspects are an integral part of the process, and enhancing your ability to strategically navigate through them. This chapter delves into these challenges, how they impact your path to habit hacking, and the strategies you can deploy to smooth your journey.

10.1. The Nature of Setbacks

It's crucial from the outset to internalize that setbacks are normal and practically inevitable. Like any journey, there will be bumps on the road, unexpected turns, and stalls. Setbacks in your habit hacking journey might be as a result of external circumstances – illness, work demands, personal crises – or internal factors, such as self-doubt, fear, lack of motivation or even temporary exhaustion from the required discipline. Understanding and acknowledging these factors can transform how setbacks impact you. It's not about never slipping or faltering, it's about getting back up and continuing the journey each time.

10.2. Developing a Resilient Mindset

Developing a resilient mindset is your first defense against setbacks. Cultivating resilience involves modifying your thought patterns to foster optimism, personal control, acceptance, and the ability to perceive adversity as an opportunity for personal growth. This mental shift can be facilitated through cognitive behavioral techniques, mindfulness practice, and meditation. There's also a growing body of research illustrating the benefits of gratitude practice for cementing resilience – consistent expression of thanks can drastically recalibrate your perspective on setbacks.

10.3. A Proactive Plan for Setbacks

Though it sounds counterintuitive, anticipating setbacks and having a proactive plan to address them can immensely lessen their impact. This might involve identifying potential pitfalls and preparing coping strategies in advance – a 'if this, then that' strategy. For instance, if a late-night work session threatens your early morning gym routine, you might plan to fit in a shorter intense home workout later in the day. If stress tempts you to resort to old habits, you might preemptively cultivate healthier stress management techniques.

10.4. Leverage Your Support Network

Don't underestimate the power of social support in overcoming setbacks. Friends, family, mentors or peers can provide necessary emotional support, remind you of your progress, offer fresh perspectives, or even give you that push when difficulties seem insurmountable. Additionally, connection with others on similar journeys can prove uniquely supportive - consider joining or forming a habit hacking support group or accountability partnership.

10.5. Reflection and Re-evaluation

Experiencing setbacks can be disheartening, but it is valuable to adopt a perspective of growth. Each time you experience a setback, consider it an occasion to pause, reflect, and learn. What were the underlying circumstances or thought patterns that led to the setback?

Do you need to adapt your strategies, environment, routine or mindset? Sometimes a setback is just a sign that your strategies need tweaking, or your goals need adjusting. They can be an essential cog in refining your habit hacking journey.

10.6. Celebrating Progress, Not Just Success

One of the easiest ways to get derailed by setbacks is to adopt a perfectionistic, 'all-or-nothing' mentality towards habit hacking. We often set ourselves rigid targets and beat ourselves up when we deviate slightly. This can sap motivation and create a cycle of repeated setbacks. Remember, the process of habit hacking involves incremental progress. You're laying one brick at a time, day by day, not building the entire wall in one go. Celebrate your progress, no matter how small, and use it as a motivation to keep moving forward despite the setbacks.

In conclusion, setbacks are a natural component of your journey towards habit hacking. They do not spell the end of your journey. Handled strategically, they can provide powerful opportunities for learning, growth, and the development of resilience. Seek to anticipate and prepare for them, leverage your support network, constantly reflect and adapt, and celebrate every stride you make, regardless the magnitude. This approach not only ensures you overcome setbacks but also reinforces the habit-forming process, making your path to success smoother and more enjoyable despite the bumps along the way.

Chapter 11. The Influence of Habit Mastery on Success: Real Life Stories

Understanding the profound impact of habit mastery on success can be made more tangible through real life stories that illustrate its efficacy. The change instigated by swapping poor habits with empowering ones has the potential to instigate monumental progress and fuel unparalleled achievements. The experiences shared in this chapter will help you apprehend the potency of good habits, providing not only inspiration, but also insights into pragmatic steps leading up to a flourishing life.

11.1. The Metamorphosis of a Best-selling Author

Imagine an aspiring writer struggling with making writing a consistent habit. James, after countless failed attempts at maintaining a regular writing schedule, decided to meticulously plan his day with dedicated writing hours. He prioritized developing this habit to fuel his literary ambitions. During the first few weeks, he showed up to write for two hours regardless of how he felt. Slowly, he began experiencing a surge in his creativity and productivity. This consistency potentiated a compound effect, and within a year, James had finished his debut novel. Now a best-selling author, he attributes his success to his disciplined habit of daily writing. In his story, we see the transformative power a deliberately cultivated habit can wield on our lives.

11.2. The Transformation of an Olympic Athlete

Another real-life parable of the power of habit mastery is the story of Rebecca, who went from being an average swimmer to an Olympic champion. When she recognized the power of habits, she built a rigorous daily routine that started with an early morning swim. Integrating this regimen took effort, willpower, and resilience, but she committed to it nevertheless, grasping its long-term potential. Her swim times accelerated remarkably, turning heads in her local swimming community, and eventually, Rebecca earned her spot in the Olympics. It wasn't inborn talent or luck that won Rebecca her shining gold medal, but her relentless pursuit of habit mastery.

11.3. The Architect of his Own Success Story

Consider the case of a Silicon Valley entrepreneur, William. He had a revolutionary idea but lacked the necessary organization and focus to bring his concept to life. He learned about the power of habits and decided to install the habit of meticulous planning and evaluation into his daily schedule. Initially, it seemed almost insurmountable, but as weeks turned into months, he successfully ingrained this habit. William also attended daily meditation practice to enhance his focus and adopted a morning reading habit to broaden his perspective. Consequently, he started making remarkable progress, and his once-struggling start-up started picking up steam. Today, his firm is among the industry leaders, validating the life-changing impact of habit formation.

To summarize, the formation of beneficial habits and breaking free from detrimental ones are vital contributors to success. Building meaningful habits requires a blend of willpower, resilience, and patience, but the reward of unlocking a more successful, productive, and balanced life makes the journey worthwhile. The stories we have explored in this chapter bear testament to the power of habit mastery. Let these stories be your beacon as you embark on your own habit-hacking expedition.

Remember, your life today is the sum total of your habits. With the right ones, you are more than capable of writing your own success story. As the progenitor of behavioral psychology, William James, once said, "All our life, so far as it has definite form, is but a mass of habits." Embrace the potent potential of your habits and witness your success soar.